FOOD DIARY

A DAILY LOG FOR WEIGHT LOSS

THIS DIET LOG BOOK BELONGS TO:

_____

DEDICATION

This Food Diary Journal Log book is dedicated to all the people out there who want to get healthier by tracking their daily food intake and document their findings in the process.

You are my inspiration for producing books and I'm honored to be a part of keeping all of your Food Diary notes and records organized.

This journal notebook will help you record your details about getting into better shape.

Thoughtfully put together with these sections to record: Daily Nutrition Log, Breakfast, Lunch, Dinner & Snacks, Daily Total and Reflection Page.

How To Use This Book:

The purpose of this book is to keep all of your Food Intake notes all in one place. It will help keep you organized.

This Food Diary Journal will allow you to accurately document every detail about tracking your daily food intake. It's a great way to chart your course to a health you.

Here are examples of the prompts for you to fill in and write about your experience in this book:

1. Daily Nutrition Log - Record & Write Fat, Calories, Sugar, Carbs, Protein, Fiber & Sodium for Meals and Snacks.

2. Breakfast, Lunch, Dinner & Snacks - Log your Food Intake for each meal you eat and snack for the day.

3. Daily Total - Keep track of your Daily Totals.

4. Reflection Page - For writing how your day went, did you exercise, water intake you consumed, activity, any symptoms you experiences, stool, weight loss amount & results, etc. or any other important information you want.

Enjoy!

Daily Nutrition Log

Breakfast	Fat	Calories

Lunch	Fat	Calories

Dinner	Fat	Calories

Snack	Fat	Calories

DATE: _____

SUGAR	CARBS	PROTEIN	FIBER	SODIUM

SUGAR	CARBS	PROTEIN	FIBER	SODIUM

SUGAR	CARBS	PROTEIN	FIBER	SODIUM

SUGAR	CARBS	PROTEIN	FIBER	SODIUM

Daily Total

Fat	
Calories	
Sugar	
Carbs	
Protein	
Fiber	
Sodium	

Notes

REFLECTION

Daily Nutrition Log

Breakfast	Fat	Calories
Lunch	Fat	Calories
Dinner	Fat	Calories
Snack	Fat	Calories

DATE: _____

SUGAR	CARBS	PROTEIN	FIBER	SODIUM

SUGAR	CARBS	PROTEIN	FIBER	SODIUM

SUGAR	CARBS	PROTEIN	FIBER	SODIUM

SUGAR	CARBS	PROTEIN	FIBER	SODIUM

DAILY TOTAL

FAT	
CALORIES	
SUGAR	
CARBS	
PROTEIN	
FIBER	
SODIUM	

NOTES

REFLECTION

Daily Nutrition Log

Breakfast	Fat	Calories

Lunch	Fat	Calories

Dinner	Fat	Calories

Snack	Fat	Calories

DATE: _____

SUGAR	CARBS	PROTEIN	FIBER	SODIUM

SUGAR	CARBS	PROTEIN	FIBER	SODIUM

SUGAR	CARBS	PROTEIN	FIBER	SODIUM

SUGAR	CARBS	PROTEIN	FIBER	SODIUM

DAILY TOTAL

FAT	
CALORIES	
SUGAR	
CARBS	
PROTEIN	
FIBER	
SODIUM	

NOTES

REFLECTION

Daily Nutrition Log

Breakfast	Fat	Calories

Lunch	Fat	Calories

Dinner	Fat	Calories

Snack	Fat	Calories

DATE: _____

SUGAR	CARBS	PROTEIN	FIBER	SODIUM

SUGAR	CARBS	PROTEIN	FIBER	SODIUM

SUGAR	CARBS	PROTEIN	FIBER	SODIUM

SUGAR	CARBS	PROTEIN	FIBER	SODIUM

DAILY TOTAL

FAT	
CALORIES	
SUGAR	
CARBS	
PROTEIN	
FIBER	
SODIUM	

NOTES

_____

_____

_____

_____

_____

_____

_____

_____

_____

REFLECTION

Daily Nutrition Log

Breakfast	Fat	Calories

Lunch	Fat	Calories

Dinner	Fat	Calories

Snack	Fat	Calories

DATE: _____

SUGAR	CARBS	PROTEIN	FIBER	SODIUM

SUGAR	CARBS	PROTEIN	FIBER	SODIUM

SUGAR	CARBS	PROTEIN	FIBER	SODIUM

SUGAR	CARBS	PROTEIN	FIBER	SODIUM

DAILY TOTAL

FAT	
CALORIES	
SUGAR	
CARBS	
PROTEIN	
FIBER	
SODIUM	

NOTES

_____

_____

_____

_____

_____

_____

_____

_____

_____

REFLECTION

Daily Nutrition Log

Breakfast	Fat	Calories

Lunch	Fat	Calories

Dinner	Fat	Calories

Snack	Fat	Calories

DATE: _____

SUGAR	CARBS	PROTEIN	FIBER	SODIUM

SUGAR	CARBS	PROTEIN	FIBER	SODIUM

SUGAR	CARBS	PROTEIN	FIBER	SODIUM

SUGAR	CARBS	PROTEIN	FIBER	SODIUM

Daily Total

Fat	
Calories	
Sugar	
Carbs	
Protein	
Fiber	
Sodium	

Notes

_____

_____

_____

_____

_____

_____

_____

_____

_____

REFLECTION

DAILY NUTRITION LOG

BREAKFAST	FAT	CALORIES

LUNCH	FAT	CALORIES

DINNER	FAT	CALORIES

SNACK	FAT	CALORIES

DATE: _____

SUGAR	CARBS	PROTEIN	FIBER	SODIUM

SUGAR	CARBS	PROTEIN	FIBER	SODIUM

SUGAR	CARBS	PROTEIN	FIBER	SODIUM

SUGAR	CARBS	PROTEIN	FIBER	SODIUM

DAILY TOTAL

FAT	
CALORIES	
SUGAR	
CARBS	
PROTEIN	
FIBER	
SODIUM	

NOTES

REFLECTION

Daily Nutrition Log

Breakfast	Fat	Calories

Lunch	Fat	Calories

Dinner	Fat	Calories

Snack	Fat	Calories

DATE: _____

SUGAR	CARBS	PROTEIN	FIBER	SODIUM

SUGAR	CARBS	PROTEIN	FIBER	SODIUM

SUGAR	CARBS	PROTEIN	FIBER	SODIUM

SUGAR	CARBS	PROTEIN	FIBER	SODIUM

DAILY TOTAL

FAT	
CALORIES	
SUGAR	
CARBS	
PROTEIN	
FIBER	
SODIUM	

NOTES

_____

_____

_____

_____

_____

_____

_____

_____

_____

REFLECTION

Daily Nutrition Log

Breakfast	Fat	Calories

Lunch	Fat	Calories

Dinner	Fat	Calories

Snack	Fat	Calories

DATE: _____

SUGAR	CARBS	PROTEIN	FIBER	SODIUM

SUGAR	CARBS	PROTEIN	FIBER	SODIUM

SUGAR	CARBS	PROTEIN	FIBER	SODIUM

SUGAR	CARBS	PROTEIN	FIBER	SODIUM

DAILY TOTAL

FAT	
CALORIES	
SUGAR	
CARBS	
PROTEIN	
FIBER	
SODIUM	

NOTES

_____

_____

_____

_____

_____

_____

_____

_____

_____

REFLECTION

Daily Nutrition Log

Breakfast	Fat	Calories

Lunch	Fat	Calories

Dinner	Fat	Calories

Snack	Fat	Calories

DATE: _____

SUGAR	CARBS	PROTEIN	FIBER	SODIUM

SUGAR	CARBS	PROTEIN	FIBER	SODIUM

SUGAR	CARBS	PROTEIN	FIBER	SODIUM

SUGAR	CARBS	PROTEIN	FIBER	SODIUM

Daily Total

Fat	
Calories	
Sugar	
Carbs	
Protein	
Fiber	
Sodium	

Notes

_____

_____

_____

_____

_____

_____

_____

_____

_____

REFLECTION

Daily Nutrition Log

Breakfast	Fat	Calories
Lunch	Fat	Calories
Dinner	Fat	Calories
Snack	Fat	Calories

DATE: _____

SUGAR	CARBS	PROTEIN	FIBER	SODIUM

SUGAR	CARBS	PROTEIN	FIBER	SODIUM

SUGAR	CARBS	PROTEIN	FIBER	SODIUM

SUGAR	CARBS	PROTEIN	FIBER	SODIUM

DAILY TOTAL

FAT	
CALORIES	
SUGAR	
CARBS	
PROTEIN	
FIBER	
SODIUM	

NOTES

REFLECTION

Daily Nutrition Log

Breakfast	Fat	Calories

Lunch	Fat	Calories

Dinner	Fat	Calories

Snack	Fat	Calories

DATE: _____

SUGAR	CARBS	PROTEIN	FIBER	SODIUM

SUGAR	CARBS	PROTEIN	FIBER	SODIUM

SUGAR	CARBS	PROTEIN	FIBER	SODIUM

SUGAR	CARBS	PROTEIN	FIBER	SODIUM

Daily Total

Fat	
Calories	
Sugar	
Carbs	
Protein	
Fiber	
Sodium	

Notes

_____

_____

_____

_____

_____

_____

_____

_____

_____

REFLECTION

DAILY NUTRITION LOG

BREAKFAST	FAT	CALORIES

LUNCH	FAT	CALORIES

DINNER	FAT	CALORIES

SNACK	FAT	CALORIES

DATE: _____

SUGAR	CARBS	PROTEIN	FIBER	SODIUM

SUGAR	CARBS	PROTEIN	FIBER	SODIUM

SUGAR	CARBS	PROTEIN	FIBER	SODIUM

SUGAR	CARBS	PROTEIN	FIBER	SODIUM

DAILY TOTAL

FAT	
CALORIES	
SUGAR	
CARBS	
PROTEIN	
FIBER	
SODIUM	

NOTES

REFLECTION

Daily Nutrition Log

Breakfast	Fat	Calories

Lunch	Fat	Calories

Dinner	Fat	Calories

Snack	Fat	Calories

DATE: _____

SUGAR	CARBS	PROTEIN	FIBER	SODIUM

SUGAR	CARBS	PROTEIN	FIBER	SODIUM

SUGAR	CARBS	PROTEIN	FIBER	SODIUM

SUGAR	CARBS	PROTEIN	FIBER	SODIUM

DAILY TOTAL

FAT	
CALORIES	
SUGAR	
CARBS	
PROTEIN	
FIBER	
SODIUM	

NOTES

_____

_____

_____

_____

_____

_____

_____

_____

_____

REFLECTION

Daily Nutrition Log

Breakfast	Fat	Calories

Lunch	Fat	Calories

Dinner	Fat	Calories

Snack	Fat	Calories

DATE: _____

SUGAR	CARBS	PROTEIN	FIBER	SODIUM

SUGAR	CARBS	PROTEIN	FIBER	SODIUM

SUGAR	CARBS	PROTEIN	FIBER	SODIUM

SUGAR	CARBS	PROTEIN	FIBER	SODIUM

Daily Total

Fat	
Calories	
Sugar	
Carbs	
Protein	
Fiber	
Sodium	

Notes

_____

_____

_____

_____

_____

_____

_____

_____

REFLECTION

Daily Nutrition Log

Breakfast	Fat	Calories

Lunch	Fat	Calories

Dinner	Fat	Calories

Snack	Fat	Calories

DATE: _____

Sugar	Carbs	Protein	Fiber	Sodium

Sugar	Carbs	Protein	Fiber	Sodium

Sugar	Carbs	Protein	Fiber	Sodium

Sugar	Carbs	Protein	Fiber	Sodium

DAILY TOTAL

FAT	
CALORIES	
SUGAR	
CARBS	
PROTEIN	
FIBER	
SODIUM	

NOTES

REFLECTION

Daily Nutrition Log

Breakfast	Fat	Calories

Lunch	Fat	Calories

Dinner	Fat	Calories

Snack	Fat	Calories

DATE: _____

SUGAR	CARBS	PROTEIN	FIBER	SODIUM

SUGAR	CARBS	PROTEIN	FIBER	SODIUM

SUGAR	CARBS	PROTEIN	FIBER	SODIUM

SUGAR	CARBS	PROTEIN	FIBER	SODIUM

Daily Total

Fat	
Calories	
Sugar	
Carbs	
Protein	
Fiber	
Sodium	

Notes

_____

_____

_____

_____

_____

_____

_____

_____

_____

REFLECTION

Daily Nutrition Log

Breakfast	Fat	Calories

Lunch	Fat	Calories

Dinner	Fat	Calories

Snack	Fat	Calories

DATE: _____

SUGAR	CARBS	PROTEIN	FIBER	SODIUM

SUGAR	CARBS	PROTEIN	FIBER	SODIUM

SUGAR	CARBS	PROTEIN	FIBER	SODIUM

SUGAR	CARBS	PROTEIN	FIBER	SODIUM

DAILY TOTAL

FAT	
CALORIES	
SUGAR	
CARBS	
PROTEIN	
FIBER	
SODIUM	

NOTES

_____

_____

_____

_____

_____

_____

_____

_____

_____

REFLECTION

Daily Nutrition Log

Breakfast	Fat	Calories

Lunch	Fat	Calories

Dinner	Fat	Calories

Snack	Fat	Calories

DATE: _____

SUGAR	CARBS	PROTEIN	FIBER	SODIUM

SUGAR	CARBS	PROTEIN	FIBER	SODIUM

SUGAR	CARBS	PROTEIN	FIBER	SODIUM

SUGAR	CARBS	PROTEIN	FIBER	SODIUM

DAILY TOTAL

FAT	
CALORIES	
SUGAR	
CARBS	
PROTEIN	
FIBER	
SODIUM	

NOTES

REFLECTION

Daily Nutrition Log

Breakfast	Fat	Calories

Lunch	Fat	Calories

Dinner	Fat	Calories

Snack	Fat	Calories

DATE: _____

Sugar	Carbs	Protein	Fiber	Sodium

Sugar	Carbs	Protein	Fiber	Sodium

Sugar	Carbs	Protein	Fiber	Sodium

Sugar	Carbs	Protein	Fiber	Sodium

DAILY TOTAL

FAT	
CALORIES	
SUGAR	
CARBS	
PROTEIN	
FIBER	
SODIUM	

NOTES

REFLECTION

Daily Nutrition Log

Breakfast	Fat	Calories

Lunch	Fat	Calories

Dinner	Fat	Calories

Snack	Fat	Calories

DATE: _____

SUGAR	CARBS	PROTEIN	FIBER	SODIUM

SUGAR	CARBS	PROTEIN	FIBER	SODIUM

SUGAR	CARBS	PROTEIN	FIBER	SODIUM

SUGAR	CARBS	PROTEIN	FIBER	SODIUM

DAILY TOTAL

FAT	
CALORIES	
SUGAR	
CARBS	
PROTEIN	
FIBER	
SODIUM	

NOTES

REFLECTION

Daily Nutrition Log

Breakfast	Fat	Calories

Lunch	Fat	Calories

Dinner	Fat	Calories

Snack	Fat	Calories

DATE: _____

SUGAR	CARBS	PROTEIN	FIBER	SODIUM

SUGAR	CARBS	PROTEIN	FIBER	SODIUM

SUGAR	CARBS	PROTEIN	FIBER	SODIUM

SUGAR	CARBS	PROTEIN	FIBER	SODIUM

DAILY TOTAL

FAT	
CALORIES	
SUGAR	
CARBS	
PROTEIN	
FIBER	
SODIUM	

NOTES

REFLECTION

Daily Nutrition Log

Breakfast	Fat	Calories

Lunch	Fat	Calories

Dinner	Fat	Calories

Snack	Fat	Calories

DATE: _____

SUGAR	CARBS	PROTEIN	FIBER	SODIUM

SUGAR	CARBS	PROTEIN	FIBER	SODIUM

SUGAR	CARBS	PROTEIN	FIBER	SODIUM

SUGAR	CARBS	PROTEIN	FIBER	SODIUM

DAILY TOTAL

FAT	
CALORIES	
SUGAR	
CARBS	
PROTEIN	
FIBER	
SODIUM	

NOTES

REFLECTION

Daily Nutrition Log

Breakfast	Fat	Calories

Lunch	Fat	Calories

Dinner	Fat	Calories

Snack	Fat	Calories

DATE: _____

SUGAR	CARBS	PROTEIN	FIBER	SODIUM

SUGAR	CARBS	PROTEIN	FIBER	SODIUM

SUGAR	CARBS	PROTEIN	FIBER	SODIUM

SUGAR	CARBS	PROTEIN	FIBER	SODIUM

DAILY TOTAL

FAT	
CALORIES	
SUGAR	
CARBS	
PROTEIN	
FIBER	
SODIUM	

NOTES

REFLECTION

Daily Nutrition Log

Breakfast	Fat	Calories

Lunch	Fat	Calories

Dinner	Fat	Calories

Snack	Fat	Calories

DATE: _____

SUGAR	CARBS	PROTEIN	FIBER	SODIUM

SUGAR	CARBS	PROTEIN	FIBER	SODIUM

SUGAR	CARBS	PROTEIN	FIBER	SODIUM

SUGAR	CARBS	PROTEIN	FIBER	SODIUM

DAILY TOTAL

FAT	
CALORIES	
SUGAR	
CARBS	
PROTEIN	
FIBER	
SODIUM	

NOTES

_____

_____

_____

_____

_____

_____

_____

_____

REFLECTION

Recipe

Title :_____

Source: _____

Cook Time: _____   Servings: _____

Ingredients

_____

_____

_____

_____

_____

_____

_____

Directions

_____

_____

_____

_____

_____

_____

_____

_____

Recipe

Title :_____

Source: _____

Cook Time: _____   Servings: _____

Ingredients

_____

_____

_____

_____

_____

_____

_____

Directions

_____

_____

_____

_____

_____

_____

_____

_____

RECIPE

TITLE :_____

SOURCE: _____

COOK TIME: _____   SERVINGS: _____

INGREDIENTS

_____

_____

_____

_____

_____

_____

_____

DIRECTIONS

_____

_____

_____

_____

_____

_____

_____

_____

RECIPE

TITLE :_____

SOURCE: _____

COOK TIME: _____ SERVINGS: _____

INGREDIENTS

_____

_____

_____

_____

_____

_____

_____

_____

DIRECTIONS

_____

_____

_____

_____

_____

_____

_____

Recipe

Title :_____

Source: _____

Cook Time: _____   Servings: _____

Ingredients

_____

_____

_____

_____

_____

_____

_____

Directions

_____

_____

_____

_____

_____

_____

_____

_____

Recipe

Title :_____

Source: _____

Cook Time: _____   Servings: _____

Ingredients

_____

_____

_____

_____

_____

_____

_____

Directions

_____

_____

_____

_____

_____

_____

_____

Recipe

Title :_____

Source: _____

Cook Time: _____   Servings: _____

Ingredients

_____

_____

_____

_____

_____

_____

_____

Directions

_____

_____

_____

_____

_____

_____

_____

Recipe

Title :_____

Source: _____

Cook Time: _____   Servings: _____

Ingredients

_____

_____

_____

_____

_____

_____

_____

_____

Directions

_____

_____

_____

_____

_____

_____

_____

_____

Recipe

Title :_____

Source: _____

Cook Time: _____   Servings: _____

Ingredients

_____

_____

_____

_____

_____

_____

_____

Directions

_____

_____

_____

_____

_____

_____

_____

www.ingramcontent.com/pod-product-compliance
Lightning Source LLC
Chambersburg PA
CBHW051028030426
42336CB00015B/2779